Natural Remedies for Reversing Gray Hair

Nutrition and Herbs for Anti-aging and Optimum Health

Thomas W. Xander

2012
Winter Tempest Books

DEDICATION

In memory of my grandparents.

CONTENTS

1 INTRODUCTION: GRAY HAIR IS A HEALTH ISSUE

According to conventional thought, gray hair is an inevitable part of aging, the amount of gray hair you have and when you get it is most likely related to genetics and there is no cure.

Furthermore, because allopathic medicine generally regards gray hair (achromotrichia) as a matter of vanity, except in cases where it is considered premature or associated with another recognized disease, no remedy is seriously pursued. When confronted with gray hair, the most common solution is to use toxic hair dyes in an attempt to cover up the problem.

But, to the alternative healer, the condition of the hair reflects the overall health of the body. Gray hair is a sign that the body is not receiving proper nutrition and is under some kind of stress, which, if left unaddressed, may lead to an overall decline in health.

There are numerous possible causes for the appearance of gray hair at any time of life, however, except in cases involving another disease, most cases of gray hair occur because of deficient nutrition. Nutritional deficiency appears to be the lone cause of gray hair, at times, and a catalyst for the secondary causes of it at other times. But, even when other factors like stress, hormones, digestive disorders and toxins are clearly factors, improper nutrition lies at the foundation of the problem.

Common Causes of Gray Hair

Alternative health recognizes stress as an emotional and physical condition that commonly precipitates the loss of melanin in hair. Also, impurities in the blood and a weakness in the kidneys may be linked with gray hair. Stress can rapidly deplete vitamins and minerals in the body, especially the B-complex vitamins. In a cyclical fashion, this depletion of nutrients can lead to further fatigue, anxiety, increased stress and hormonal imbalances.

The following is a break down of the common causes of gray hair:

Adrenal Fatigue is caused by extreme or prolonged stress. Such chronic stress, as well as acute stress involved in life-changing events such as moving from one place to another and changes of altitude, is known to have a tangible impact on hair health. Symptoms of adrenal fatigue may include complete and utter exhaustion along with graying, lack-luster and thinning hair. Pantothenic acid (B-5) is often lacking in these cases and certain foods, in particular, onions help restore balance.

Thyroid imbalance is frequently cited as an underlying cause of gray hair. The thyroid is the key gland responsible for hormone regulation. When it is out of balance, this is called hyperthyroidism or hypothyroidism These imbalances may be brought on by stress, pregnancy, menopause and exposure to a toxic environment and may not only be implicated in gray hair, but adversely affect the body, mind and emotions. In alternative health practices, these imbalances are remedied with nutrition and extracts from dulse kelp.

Toxic burden from heavy metals can block nutrition, interfere with cell electro-conductivity and wreak havoc on all of the tissues and organs of the body. Toxins can come from contaminated food, water, air and pharmaceutical drugs. Among these toxins are heavy and soft metals, which block the proper functioning of all of the cells in the body, including those of the blood, skin, follicles and hair.

Poor circulation causes an improper flow of blood and oxygen, which deprives the cells of the nutrients required for maintenance and repair. Circulation of the scalp may be increased through the use of topical remedies and ingesting increased amounts of oxygenating nutrients.

Vitiligo is a medically recognized disease that, by some estimates, affects about 3% of the population. It is characterized by patches of white skin and is most noticeable on those with darker skin tones. The melanin of skin and hair at those sites is depleted, which causes them to become white. Vitiligo is a particular disease of which gray hair is only one symptom, however, it is included here because the remedies for vitiligo are similar to those employed for the common condition of gray hair.

Nutritional deficiencies are the underlying cause of most cases of gray hair, although which nutrients the body is deficient in vary. In cases where anemia is the underlying cause, increases of iron and Vitamin B12 may correct the problem. In cases where digestive enzymes are lacking, raw foods may supply the remedy. In other cases, nutritional deficiencies contribute to imbalances in the system, digestive disorders or a large toxic burden. Changing the diet, eliminating certain foods and including certain other foods may remedy the situation.

Aging is considered to be a cause of gray hair, which is accepted by the mainstream mindset as a fait accompli. Interestingly, besides bringing nutrition into balance, many gray hair remedies, also, have rejuvenating and anti-aging properties. So, pursuing a personal solution to the problem of gray hair often leads people to an overall improvement in appearance and the return of their youthful vigor.

Other causes frequently cited, correctly or incorrectly, in the condition of gray hair are heredity, smoking, chronic sinusitus, washing the hair with hot water, drying with an electric dryer, the use of chemical hair dyes and harsh, detergent shampoos containing sodium lauryl (or laureth) sulfate, a substance which is damaging to hair follicles.

How to Use the Information in this Book

Neither the cause nor the remedy is the same for every person with gray hair. So, to find the solution to your personal gray hair problem, you will have to do a little self-assessment. Examine your own dietary habits and determine which ones you want to include and which ones you want to eliminate.

Your body has an intelligence all its own, so listen to your intuition and to your body's cravings. Very often when the body is deficient in a particular nutrient, it will crave the very foods that will help to remedy the problem. As you go through the information in this book, pay attention to those nutrients you feel you might be lacking in. Take notice if a particular remedy resonates with you and make a note of this.

As you go through the remedies, you will observe that many of them which have strong claims of hair reversal frequently have very similar nutritional properties. Typically, these are Vitamins A, B-complex, C, E and the four minerals copper, zinc, magnesium and manganese. Iodine-containing herbs and living enzymes, also, play a role in many of them.

A remarkably accurate way to let your body tell you what it needs is through the use of medical radiesthesia. More information about radiesthesia is given in the book, *Magical Healing: How to Use Your Mind to Heal Yourself and Others*, by Angela Kaelin, an extract from which, along with an exercise adapted to the gray hair remedies presented herein, can be found in the last chapter of this book. This can be approached both as a fun experiment and a way to determine which nutrients or remedies to include in your personal gray hair reversal regimen.

Please, keep in mind that all of gray hair remedies take weeks and sometimes two or three months to produce noticeable results. So, commitment and patience is required along with persistence. If a remedy does not produce a good result after about three months, its probably the wrong remedy for you and you should try another one. You may, also, wish to employ multiple remedies at a time. Typically, a combination of diet, supplements and a topical remedy are employed together.

Abbreviation Key

T. = Tablespoon
tsp. = teaspoon
g = gram
mg = milligrams

Conversion of Measurements

3 tsp. = 1 T.
1 tsp. = approximately 4.2 g
1 cup liquid = approximately 220 to 240 g
1 cup non-liquid = approximately 120 to140 g
1 g = 1000 mg
1 mg = 0.001 grams

2 THE BASIC ANTI-GRAY HAIR DIET

Alternative healers define good health as the optimal functioning of the body and all of its organs and cells. Disease is seen as the result of an imbalance in the body. When there is a sign that something in the body is malfunctioning (such as the cessation of melanin production in hair cells), the alternative healer looks for the cause of the imbalance and tries to find a remedy to bring the body's system back into harmony.

A major cause of illness in the West is the modern diet, which is woefully deficient of nutrients and laden with toxins that weaken the body's cells and open the door to a variety of diseases.

Proper nutrition helps the body to expel toxins from the tissues and fortifies your body so that it can fight disease and aging. A healthy diet should be the foundation to which you add your anti-gray hair regimen.

Many of the following suggestions are common knowledge, but it is necessary to comment on them because no matter which gray hair remedies you decide to try, it is important to have a good basic diet at the foundation of your efforts.

What to Include

Because of the allopathic belief in Germ Theory, which is the notion that disease is caused by the spread of germs, food is sterilized by heat pasteurization, radiation or chemical processes, which alters the food, depletes the nutritional value, destroys the healthy bacteria and enzymes required for proper digestion and renders it unhealthy and unsafe. For example, raw dairy products heal the body while pasteurized dairy products are associated with the formation of tumors, allergies, lactose intolerance and other diseases.

Therefore, whenever possible choose raw dairy, honey, fruits and vegetables instead of pasteurized and processed versions of these foods. Raw, unpasteurized foods contain living enzymes that processed foods do not. These components of living food provide cells with the nutrition they need to repair and fortify themselves.

While it is important to eat plenty of fresh, raw fruits and vegetables, the best way to obtain the most pure, rich nutrients from them is through the use of a high-quality juicer. Freshly made juices contain living enzymes necessary for digestion and to help strengthen and detoxify the cells and organs of the body.

As much as possible, eat at home and create meals from scratch. Make soups from scratch using your own homemade broth and include tissue from the bones, the marrow, joints and cartilage. Avoid processed food, frozen dinners and fast food, which is often laden with high levels of sodium chloride, excitotoxins (flavor enhancers like MSG), preservatives and other unwholesome ingredients. By contrast, eating soups from homemade broth helps provide the body with the nutrients for all of the tissues of the body including the hair follicles.

What to Avoid

Avoid artificial ingredients in fast food, processed foods and beverages, such as the following:

Artificial sweeteners such as apsartame and sucralose are linked to a variety of neurological disorders and diseases, as well as hair loss.

Aspartame is considered by some experts to be the most dangerous of all food additives, however, it is permitted in foods in the U.S. It is sold under many different names, including NutraSweet and Equal, and is found in most brands of chewing gum and a surprising number of foods and beverages, even those that contain sugar. Even if you are carefully reading labels, you may not realize that aspartame is in the product.

Aspartame metabolizes as methanol (toxic wood alcohol) in the body and converts into formaldehyde (used in embalming), which lodges in the brain tissues. Among other things, it destroys healthy intestinal flora required for proper digestion.

Sucralose is a sugar molecule with one of the ions altered to chlorine. It is sold under the trade name Splenda and is found in a surprising number of commercially prepared products and even some public water supplies. In tests on lab rats, it caused a large reduction in the size of the thymus gland and enlargement of the liver and kidneys. The improper function of these organs may lead to gray hair.

Despite the fact that artificial sweeteners like aspartame and sucralose may be dangerous and addictive, allopathic medical doctors commonly recommend them as a sugar substitute to their patients who suffer from diabetes. Although, there are healthier substitutes, particularly coconut sugar, which is highly nutritious and has a warm, natural taste similar to unprocessed raw sugar. According to the Food and Nutrition Research Institute (FNRI) of the Department of Science and Technology (DOST) of The Philippines, coconut sugar is considered safe for diabetics because of its very low glycemic index of 35. [1]

Consuming artificial sweeteners is counterproductive to any gray hair reversal regimen because of their harmful side effects and lack of nutritional value. By contrast, natural sweeteners like raw honey, raw sugar and coconut sugar all provide important nutritional support to the body.

High fructose corn syrup is another sweetener found in all kinds of beverages, particularly sodas and processed foods. It is linked to heart disease, obesity, cancer, dementia, liver failure and it contains contaminants like mercury, which is associated with hair graying and hair loss.

Consuming high fructose corn syrup depletes the body's supply of digestive enzymes, vitamins and minerals, including magnesium and copper, which are vital to the production of melanocytes necessary to maintain the natural color of hair.

MSG (monosodium glutamate) is a flavor enhancer that goes by a remarkable of number of names (ie. natural flavoring and hydrolyzed vegetable protein, maltodextrin, etc.) and appears in many processed foods, including infant formulas and restaurant-prepared foods, most notoriously Chinese food.

According to Dr. Russell L. Blaylock, M.D., in his book, Excitotoxins: The Taste That Kills, MSG is an excitotoxin, which agitates brain cells to death.[2] It contributes to obesity, cardiovascular and other diseases and binds with aspartame in the system to form a toxic compound.

Sodium fluoride is found in tap water, some brands of drinking water, most commercial toothpastes and many mouthwashes. It is not fluorine, which is a naturally occurring trace mineral, vital to human health. Instead, sodium fluoride is a fluorine mimicker and when insufficient amounts of fluorine are present in the system, the body will absorb this toxin into the tissues.

To avoid sodium fluoride, drink and cook with distilled water. Tap water presents other dangers in the form of toxic chemicals like chlorine, which is misguidedly added to the water to purify it, along with the residue of pharmaceutical drugs which can be very harmful to overall health.

Choose more natural dentifrices. Old-fashioned lye soap made from lye and tallow makes and excellent substitute for toothpaste and there are plenty of healthier ways to cleanse the entire mouth, including oil pulling and rinsing with pure colloidal silver.

Common table salt (sodium chloride) is used in restaurant-prepared foods and many processed foods. It is an unsafe chemical compound created by the process of extracting the salt from mines, during which many of the beneficial minerals and nutrients are stripped from it. It is associated with unhealthy, thinning hair.

Himalayan salt and sea salt from evaporated sea water are healthier alternatives, because they retain their natural, rich mineral content. Some people have reported positive changes in their hair color by using mineral rich Himalayan salt.

Cravings for salt may be the body telling you that it has a low-functioning thyroid due to a deficiency of iodine.

As always, if you are under the care of a physician consult with him or her before making any changes in your diet.

3 DETOXIFYING REGIMEN
FOR GRAY HAIR REVERSAL

Try as we might, it is impossible to completely eliminate all of the toxins from our diet because they are now present virtually everywhere on the planet, in the air, soil and water. This is why it is important to use a detoxifying remedy along with good nutrition to help our bodies expel these poisons.

Oil pulling is an ancient Indian method of cleaning the mouth and healing the gums and teeth, which provides overall detoxifying benefits to the body. Some people who have used this technique alone have seen their hair begin to return to its natural color in a matter of several weeks.

Any of the following oils can be used:

Sunflower (traditionally used)
Sesame seed (traditionally used)
Apricot
Castor oil
Coconut, preferably organic, virgin

Grape seed
Hemp seed
Olive
Safflower oil

Hold approximately one tablespoon of oil in your mouth for 10 or 15 minutes. Take care not to swallow any of the oil, which will contain toxins and bacteria pulled from your tissues. Then, spit the oil into the toilet. Optionally, you may rinse your mouth with warm sea salt water. Then drink plenty of distilled water (two or three glasses) to help facilitate the removal of toxins from your entire system.

Oil pulling can be performed any time of day. Although, it is ideal to perform oil pulling upon awakening in the morning before you have anything to drink. Once per day is often enough, however, if you want to detoxify more quickly, do oil pulling two to three times per day.

Do not swallow the oil. If you happen to swallow a little bit of it and feel nauseated, place one or two drops of peppermint oil on your tongue or sip a little pineapple juice to quell the nausea.

4 VITAMINS

A deficiency of certain vitamins is often associated with gray hair. While it is important to try to get as many of these vitamins from natural food sources, this is not always possible. So, it is important to use a high quality supplement along with your vitamin-rich diet.

Vitamin A (retinol) is supportive to the health of all of the tissues of the body and the hair. It is most commonly found in orange and yellow vegetables. Good sources include beef liver, broccoli, butternut squash, mangoes, sweet potatoes, pumpkins and tomatoes. Raw, fresh carrot juice is an excellent source of Vitamin A and a well-known liver detoxifier.

B-complex vitamins are required by the body, especially when it is under high stress. Any time stress is a factor, the depletion of B-complex vitamins occurs, which leads to feelings of exhaustion and a downward spiral of health.

It is often reported that the onset of the first gray hairs are precipitated by a stressful event which can deplete the body of these nutrients, upset the adrenals and create hormonal and other imbalances in the body. The quickest way to get the body's required levels of these vitamins is through the use of supplements.

The following are critical B-vitamins and other nutrients vital to the maintenance of natural hair color and their common, natural sources:

Vitamin B1 (thiamine) from fresh peas, spinach, sunflower seeds and watermelons

Vitamin B2 (riboflavin) from broccoli, mushrooms, spinach, clams and oysters

Vitamin B3 (niacin or niacinamide) from potatoes, spinach, tomatoes, beef, tuna and shrimp

Vitamin B5 (pantothenic acid) from raw vegetables, beef, beans, liver, mushrooms, nuts and sea fish.

Vitamin B6 (pyridoxine) from acorn squash, bananas, spinach, tomatoes and watermelons

Vitamin B7 (biotin) from raw, leafy vegetables, mushrooms, brewer's yeast, beef, salmon and tuna

Vitamin B9 (folic acid) from beef liver and spinach

Vitamin B12 from fish, meat, milk and poultry

Inositol from brewer's yeast, unsulphered blackstrap molasses, wheat germ, liver and vegetables

Choline from from butter, potatoes, sesame seeds and flax

PABA (para-aminobenzoic acid) from brewer's yeast,

blackstrap molasses, spinach, whole grains and liver

Vitamin C is supplied by citrus fruits and tomatoes. It helps oxygenate the body and facilitates circulation.

Vitamin E is obtained from avocados, cod, olive oil, sunflower oil, other healthy plant oils, sweet potatoes, shrimp and wheat germ. It is vital to healthy hair and tissues.

The vitamins associated with reversal of common gray hair conditions may help with vitiligo, as well. A study by Montes, Diaz and Garcia of the Department of Dermatology, University of Alabama, Birmingham Medical Center [3] and another by Juhlin and Olson of the Department of Dermatology, University Hospital, Uppsala, Sweden [4] suggest that an addition of B9 (folic acid) and B12 together with either Vitamin C or very brief UVB ray exposure leads to an improvement in the condition.

Other studies have been done involving the PABA and vitiligo with results similar to those described above for cases of common gray hair. PABA can, also, be used as a topical agent in cases of vitiligo. Be advised that some people are allergic to PABA, including its topical form.

Stress is a precipitating and aggravating factor in cases of gray hair, including vitiligo, which is why a high-quality B-complex vitamin, including folic acid, along with 2,000 mg of Vitamin C may be particularly beneficial.

Thomas W. Xander

5 MINERALS

A deficiency of minerals is commonly cited as a suspected cause of gray hair, in particular magnesium and the trace minerals copper, manganese and zinc. These four minerals are found in the following foods and herbs.

Magnesium: Almonds, basil, blackstrap molasses, bran (rice, wheat and oat), brazil nuts, broccoli, cashews, cilantro (coriander), chives, dill, flax, mullein, nettles, primrose, pumpkin seeds, sesame seeds, spearmint and sunflower seeds.

Copper: Baby bella mushrooms (crimini mushrooms), barley, black pepper, blackstrap molasses, cashews, chickpeas, dandelion, devil's bit, leafy greens, liverwort, nuts, oysters, salep, sesame seeds, sheep sorrel and sunflower seeds.

Manganese: Blackstrap molasses, burdock, clams, cloves, kelp, hazelnuts, mussels, oysters, pecans, pine nuts, pumpkin seeds, saffron, sesame seeds, sheep's sorrel, yellow dock, and wheat germ.

Zinc: Beef, blackstrap molasses, horsetail, liver, oysters, paprika, peanuts, sesame seeds, shepherd's purse and wheat germ.

The above mentioned herbs may be taken daily in the form of a teas or tinctures. Bitter herbs like yellow dock and dandelion are more easily consumed as tinctures. Other herbs and foods such as nettles, kelp and black pepper can be added to your homemade soup and other recipes.

There are no agreed upon amounts for daily consumption of these minerals as supplements, although government recommended levels of magnesium are between approximately 300 and 400 mg daily for an adult and the others are usually taken in very tiny amounts. For example: Copper approximately 2 mg; manganese approximately 2 to 3 mg; and zinc approximately 15 mg.

Blackstrap Molasses

Unsulphured blackstrap molasses, extracted from pure, unrefined sugar cane, is a good source for all of the previously mentioned minerals, as well as iron and most of the vitamins previously cited in gray hair reversal, including B12. It is a very helpful remedy for anemia, which is sometimes believed to be a cause of gray hair.

To reverse gray hair, a person usually takes two to three tablespoons of unsulphured blackstrap molasses per day. A few people report good results with just blackstrap molasses.

But, more often, blackstrap molasses alone is not enough and it is combined into other remedies and supplement regimens.

Note: Blackstrap molasses has a glycemic index of 55. It may not be a good remedy for diabetics because it is sugar.

Regimen #1 Blackstrap Molasses
Anti-gray Hair Drink

2 to 3 T. unsulphured blackstrap molasses
2 to 3 T. raw apple cider vinegar (unpasteurized, with the mother)
1,000 to 2,000 mg wheat germ
2,000 mg brewer's yeast

Regimen #2 Blackstrap Molasses
Anti-gray Hair Drink

2 to 3 T. unsulphured blackstrap molasses
2 to 3 T. raw apple cider vinegar (unpasteurized, with the mother)
2 T. lemon juice
1 T. raw honey
1/8 tsp. fresh, ground black pepper
1/4 cup hot, distilled water

Regimen #3 Blackstrap Molasses
Anti-gray Hair Drink

1 to 2 T. blackstrap molasses
1 T. raw honey
2 T. raw apple cider vinegar
2 to 4 T. lemon juice

Take these ingredients together or separately. If you combine molasses with honey, add approximately 1/4 cup of warm water to make it easier to swallow.

Regimen #4 Blackstrap Molasses, Vitamin and Mineral Combination

2 to 3 T. unsulphured blackstrap molasses
100 mg. zinc
Vitamin B7 (Biotin)

Consume daily.

Regimen #5 Blackstrap Molasses pH Balancing

Properly balanced pH levels facilitate proper digestion and absorption of the vitamins and minerals in your food and supplements.

The formula given here is a modification of the Moreless Protocol, which once appeared on the web. The original protocol, also, included recommendations for a sensible diet consisting largely of fresh fruits and vegetables. This formula has been augmented to include two common anti-gray hair herbs, turmeric and ginger, which were not in the original.

This is an energizing, mineralizing and pH balancing drink, which has been reported to increase overall vitality and have the side effect of returning gray hair to its natural color. The purpose of the following formula is to increase the bio-availability of minerals and restore the body's natural state of electro-conductivity.

1 T. unsulphured blackstrap molasses
1 tsp. powdered kelp (or 2 to 4 drops of Heritage Products Sea-Adine or Lugol's Iodine)
1 T. lemon juice (or 1 T. raw, unpasteurized apple cider vinegar)
1 to 4 T. pickling lime water (calcium hydroxide)
A pinch of organic Epsom salts (magnesium sulfate)

1/4 cup warm distilled water
1/2 tsp. ground turmeric
1/2 tsp ground ginger

Pickling lime powder is usually available in the canning and preserving section of your local grocery store. Make the pickling lime water by adding one tablespoon of the powder to one gallon of pure, distilled water.

The first two ingredients may be included in the drink or taken separately. Combine the ingredients in a glass and dissolve the Epsom salts. Increase the amount of lemon juice and pickling lime to your liking. Take this remedy two to three times per day.

Caution: Do not inhale the powdered pickling lime. Turmeric is a natural anti-coagulant. Several pharmaceutical drugs can interact with turmeric, including Coumadin. As always, if you are under the care of a physician, consult with your doctor before taking herbs or embarking on a dietary change.

Iodine

Iodine is another important gray-hair reversing mineral. It is used to regulate the body's key adrenal gland, the thyroid.

A malfunction of the thyroid, which secretes necessary hormones, is frequently cited as the cause of gray hair. These imbalances of the thyroid gland are described as either under-functioning (hypothyroidism) or over-functioning (hyperthyroidism).

Some possible symptoms of an under-functioning thyroid (hypothyroidism) are: Slow heart rate (bradycardia); shortness of breath; weight gain; chest pains; brittle nails; dry skin; muscular cramps; chronic constipation; menstrual problems; headaches; migraines;

sinus infections; post-nasal drip; visual disturbances; swollen thyroid gland; goiter; swelling joints followed by joint pain; intolerance for cold and cold hands and feet. It is associated with Hashimoto's disease; tumors and inflammation in the thyroid gland. This condition is estimated to be about four times more common in women than men.

Some possible symptoms of an over-functioning thyroid (hyperthyroidism) are: Hair loss; rashes; fast heart rate (tachycardia); heart palpitations; shortness of breath; nervousness; tremors of the hands and feet; goiter; insomnia; weakness; increased perspiration; intolerance for heat and sudden weight loss accompanied by an increased appetite. It is associated with Grave's disease, diabetes and auto-immune disorders.

Both of these conditions cause fatigue and symptoms often associated with aging, including graying, dry, brittle, thinning hair.

The main remedy for thyroid imbalances, which, also, reverses gray hair for some people, is iodine from foods, herbs and supplements.

Where hypothyroidism (under-functioning) is suspected, levels of iodine are increased with natural sources such as fish, yogurt, meat, parsley, white (Irish) potatoes with the skins, oatmeal, bananas, mustard, kelp, dulse, sea wrack and nettles.

Where hyperthyroidism (over-functioning) is suspected, common remedies include algae, kelp, dulse, nori, coconut oil, bugle weed (lycopus europaeus L.) and lemon balm (melissa officianalis).

Kelp tablets taken in fairly high amounts provide many of the vitamins and minerals associated with gray hair reversal, including PABA.

Irish moss is, also, an excellent source of iodine. It contains Vitamins A and E along with necessary minerals and essential fatty acids.

Lugol's iodine drops and Heritage Products' Sea-Adine are popular remedies for regulating the thyroid. They should only be taken only as directed on the bottle. Taking too much can cause further imbalances.

Thyroid imbalances are associated with stress, so any protocol for this condition should, also, include remedies to help the body cope with stress, such as the B-complex vitamins. It is, also, important to drink and prepare meals with pure, preferably distilled water because tap water may be a source of thyroid-harming contaminants. Radioactive iodides have been found in some municipal water supplies in the U.S.

There are, also, increasing concerns about the possibility of fish, in particular, being contaminated with radiation since recent leaks in France, Japan and the United States. Natural dulse kelp, Irish moss and other seaweed are the classic remedies to protect the thyroid gland from such radiation, which we must become more conscious of worldwide since radiation leaks do not remain localized. Furthermore, the effects of radiation do not quickly dissipate, rather they bio-accumulate in the soil and in the tissues of animals and man.

Caution: Always follow the directions on the label of your organic, kelp-based iodine product. Only use oral iodine supplements from organic food sources, not the toxic, topical iodine available at most pharmacies, which is for external use only.

Thomas W. Xander

6 DIGESTIVE ENZYMES

Gray hair is sometimes attributed to poor digestion, which may be caused by a lack of enzymes in the food we eat. Enzymes are a living protein produced by cells. They are found in raw, unprocessed food and produced by the body.

But, as people age, the amount of natural enzymes in their digestive tract lessens, making it more difficult for their bodies to extract vital nutrients from the food they eat. Furthermore, enzymes are destroyed when food is cooked, processed or irradiated. Most people's diets are filled with food that lacks the living enzymes the body requires to properly digest it.

There are two main ways to go about getting the live enzymes you need. You may obtain them from supplements that provide these enzymes, which are available from health food stores. And, you may obtain them naturally by including living, raw and fermented foods in your diet.

Some people have experienced a complete reversal of gray hair just by switching to an entirely raw food diet.

Even if you don't want to go that far, raw foods are an important element in your gray hair reversal regimen.

Enzymes from Raw Foods

Eating whole, raw foods is an important part of an anti-gray hair diet, but the best way to get large amounts of bio-available enzymes and other nutrients you need is through juicing. You'll get the most out of your juicing experience if you use a high-quality, stainless steel constructed juicer.

Organic vegetables and those you grow yourself or purchase from small local farmers are often fresher and more nutritious than those purchased at big supermarkets.

The following raw foods may be especially helpful for providing living enzymes to the body and reversing gray hair:

Beets
Cabbage
Carrots
Celery
Chia seeds (a stand-alone remedy for some cases of gray hair)
Celery
Daikon radishes
Dark leafy green vegetables
Fenugreek seed sprouts (a stand-alone remedy for some cases of gray hair)
White (Irish) potatoes (provide the enzyme catalase, a deficiency of which is implicated in gray hair)
Sour apples including the peeling (also, provide catalase)
Wheatgrass (a stand-alone remedy, which contains many anti-gray hair vitamins and minerals)
Mulberries (a kidney tonic)

All fruits and dark berries
Raw honey, bee propolis and royal jelly

Enzymes from Raw Dairy Products

Raw milk, buttermilk, cheese, yogurt, butter and other natural products, which have been properly handled and not pasteurized or homogenized, contain the living enzymes necessary for digestion and provide overall health benefits.

Eating raw dairy products with the enzymes makes them digestible. Lactose intolerance occurs because the digestive system lacks the proper enzymes to digest dairy products because those living proteins were destroyed by the pasteurization process.

Presently, in the U.S. where forced pasteurization has been declared the law of the land, there is a war on raw dairy products that parallels the war on drugs, so you may have difficulty obtaining them from the usual sources, such as grocery stores or even farmer's markets. Co-ops have been the main targets of sometimes violent Federal raids. In many other parts of the world there are restrictions and bans. It may still be possible to obtain raw dairy products directly from farms and sometimes at grocery stores depending on the country you live in.

Enzymes from Fermented Foods

Some kind of fermented food should be part of an anti-gray hair daily diet because it both helps balance pH and aides digestion by providing digestive enzymes.

Foods beneficial to gray hair reversal are as follows:

Apple cider vinegar with the mother is full of necessary enzymes. It helps to detoxify the body, balances pH levels and aides digestion.For gray hair reversal, try two tablespoons of raw apple cider vinegar with one tablespoon of raw honey every day.

Kombucha tea is a fermented drink that is most beneficial when you brew it yourself. Kombucha colonies and instructions are available from online herb shops like The Happy Herbalist. This natural, fermented probiotic is full of amino acids and enzymes which are associated with longevity and some cases of gray hair reversal.

Miso (soybean curd) is available at many Asian groceries and some health food stores. It makes an excellent base for seaweed soup recipes.

Yogurt is a fermented dairy product. Look for raw, organic yogurt wherever possible.

Kefir is a fermented dairy drink. It is more difficult to find in the U.S. because of the pasteurization laws, consequently many people obtain kefir grains from health food stores and make it at home. It is an economical way to get digestive enzymes and probiotics into the diet.

Sourdough breads are best when they are homemade with a fermented starter and preferably whole grains.

7 ESSENTIAL FATTY ACIDS

Essential fatty acids are necessary for the health of all of your cells, but the body does not manufacture them, so they must come from the food you eat, primarily fish, grains, seeds and nuts. At least, one to two tablespoons (approximately 14 to 28 grams) of essential fatty acids, including Omega 3 and Omega 6, per day may help with gray hair reversal, anti-aging and promote healthy cell function.

The following are sources of these essential fatty acids, which are most commonly used for gray hair reversal:

Black seed oil (black cumin or nigella sativa): A legendary Indian anti-gray hair remedy

Chia seeds: A superfood credited with anti-aging and overall all health benefits

Flax seed (crushed or oil): An excellent source of

essential fatty acids

Fish oil: Omega 3 from salmon, pollock, catfish and tuna

Sesame seeds: A well-known Chinese anti-gray hair remedy

Seaweed (algae, dulse, Irish moss, nori, etc.)

Wheat germ oil: Contains high levels of Vitamin E

DHA (decosahexanoic acid): From whole grains, brown rice and oatmeal

   Note: Flax seed oil must be refrigerated and should not be heated in cooking.

8 BLOOD AND KIDNEY TONICS

The condition of the blood and kidneys is reflected in the hair. A key to graying hair is the purification of the blood and the strengthening of the kidneys.

The following foods act as tonics to the blood, kidneys or both, as indicated in parentheses:

Asparagus (kidneys)

Beets (blood)

Carrots (blood)

Blackstrap molasses (both)

Black sesame seeds (both)

Chlorophyll (both)

Cranberries (kidneys)

Cucumbers (blood)

Dandelion roots (kidneys)

Hyssop (blood)

Nettles (both)

Parsley (kidneys)

Seaweed (both)

Strawberry leaves (blood)

Watermelon seeds as a tea (kidneys)

Wheatgrass (both)

There are no pre-determined daily amounts for these unless they are described as such on the packaging. These foods and herbs can be added to the diet through juicing and as teas, decoctions and tinctures, which is the best choice in the case of bitter herbs like dandelion roots and hyssop. Seaweed, nettles, and parsley are good ingredients for soups. Beets, carrots, cucumbers and wheatgrass are highly beneficial as raw juices.

Chlorophyll

Chlorophyll is a green pigmentation found in plants. It has a similar molecular structure to hemoglobin, which plays a vital role in the proper functionality of red blood cells, facilitating oxygenation and circulation. It is regarded as a blood purifier and a heavy metals detoxifier. It contains most of the vitamins and minerals commonly associated with gray hair reversal, including

Vitamins A, B-complex, C, E and the minerals copper, magnesium, manganese and zinc.

Liquid chlorophyll extract is available from health food stores. Look for high quality and strength in these products. Taking 1/2 ounce of chlorophyll three times per day may reverse some cases of gray hair. It may, also, be helpful in cases of thinning hair and balding. Look for results after approximately three weeks.

The following is another chlorophyll remedy: Take 2,000 mg of Vitamin C with 1 T. chlorophyll from alfalfa daily.

Wheatgrass

Wheatgrass is very high in chlorophyll, as well as Vitamins A, B-complex, C and E. Wheatgrass, also, contains nearly 90% of the minerals from soil required by the body, including magnesium and zinc. All of these are vital to healthy, non-gray hair.

As previously mentioned, fresh wheatgrass may be juiced. Powdered wheatgrass may, also, be added to your juice, other beverages or food.

It is one of the most valued herbs in gray hair reversal. In some cases of gray hair, consuming wheatgrass alone is credited with bringing results in two to three weeks.

Thomas W. Xander

9 OTHER HERBS AND FOODS

Irish (White) Potatoes and Catalase

One of the most economical and delicious gray hair remedies is the common white potato, also, called the Irish potato. This remedy, which was given by Edgar Cayce, seems to be supported by a research study that revealed a correlation between the absence of the enzyme catalase and the graying of hair. Edgar Cayce's remedy involves the skins of the potato. He, also, mentions eating the peelings from citrus fruits in conjunction with potato skins to reverse gray hair.[5]

The following is based on Cayce's Irish potato remedy: Choose two medium-sized white potatoes and, essentially, make a tea from the skins. Remove the skins and boil them in water for approximately 12 minutes. You may wrap them in Patapar paper (a 100% vegetable oil cooking parchment, which does not contain silicon) to help preserve the nutrients. Allow them to cool before eating them. Add sea salt and black pepper to the potato water and drink it. Performed once or twice daily, you may begin to see a difference in a few weeks or months.

Cayce gave several different versions of this potato skin remedy to several patients. One, also, included the use of a topical oil treatment in conjunction with eating the boiled potato skins and their liquid. Some readings, also, called for the consumption of citrus fruits, which contain high amounts of Vitamin C.

Since potatoes contain high amounts of the enzyme catalase, it seems as if Cayce's potato remedy may have scientific support. According to a study conducted by the Clinical and Experimental Dermatology/Department of Biomedical Sciences, University of Bradford in the U.K., catalase is absent in the follicles of gray hairs.

The body's production of catalase decreases with age, leaving hair follicles unable to produce sufficient melanin to overcome the natural hydrogen peroxide in the body, leading to the graying of hair. An insufficient amount of catalase impedes the body's ability to breakdown hydrogen peroxide into water and oxygen, which is required for the maintenance of melanin in the hair. Furthermore, gray hair is not an entirely benign condition because this excess of hydrogen peroxide may, also, lead to cell damage.[6]

Resveratol and Catalase Production

Some people claim that taking fairly high doses of resveratrol, the red wine extract associated with longevity, has reversed their gray hair.

This claim seems to be bolstered by a research story conducted at the University of Padova in Italy in which guinea pigs, given resveratrol experienced increased production of the enzyme catalase.[7]

A minimum of 100 mg twice per day is suggested for reversing gray hair.

Lemons

Lemons provide a large number of necessary enzymes, along with Vitamin C. They help balance the body's pH levels and improve digestion. They, also, mimic hydrochloric acid in the body, a deficiency of which is associated with graying of hair.

Wash and eat lemons raw, drink the juice and eat the peelings daily as part of your anti-gray hair regimen.

Onions

Onions are a powerful anti-aging food. They are an excellent remedy for people who have been subjected to abnormal stress levels because they provide support to exhausted adrenal glands. They help to to balance the blood sugar, lower blood pressure and decrease food cravings. Eat onions daily as part of your hair reversal regimen and enjoy the benefits of increased energy.

Onions can be included in salads, soups and other recipes.

A simple recipe for the non-gourmet is to sauté a whole, white onion and a clove of garlic in a tablespoon of olive or sunflower oil. Season with salt, pepper and a dash of Worcestershire sauce.

Caution: Onions are a natural blood-thinner.

Chia Seeds

Chia seeds are an ancient Mexican crop, which has enjoyed a modern revival because of its remarkably high nutritional content. Chia seeds are mainly black or brownish gray and some are white (chia alba). While all chia seeds are considered a superfood, the white chia alba seeds have slightly more nutrients than the others.

Chia seeds are a powerful anti-oxidant, credited with

longevity and anti-aging powers. They contain Omega 3 and Omega 6 fatty acids along with the vitamins and minerals commonly implicated in graying hair, including Vitamins B, C and E and the minerals copper, magnesium, manganese and zinc.

Like flax seeds, they must be ground or chewed for the nutrients to be released. They are used in a variety of recipes, including breads, soups, salads and may be juiced and added to smoothies. They have a pleasant nutty flavor and are commonly eaten plain. Cold pressed chia seed oil is, also, available at some health food stores and online.

A typical serving of chia seeds is 15 grams, however, 1 to 3 T. daily is suggested to facilitate gray hair reversal. The daily consumption of chia seeds alone has been credited by some people with the maintenance of their natural hair color.

10 ASIAN REMEDIES

Amla (Indian gooseberry, emblica officinalis or emblic myrobalanor) is commonly regarded as a rejuvenating tonic in India. Among its many health benefits, it contains high amounts of Vitamin C and other vitamins and minerals, is a nerve tonic and supports the tissues of the body, including the hair follicles. It is credited with the maintenance of natural color and delayng the onset of gray hair. It can be used as a dry powder, fresh juice, crushed or grated.

Black seed (nigella or black cumin) oil alone is a remedy for gray hair. Take 1 tsp. per day. Optionally, combine it with 1 T. raw honey.

Black sesame seeds are common in Japan and China where they are well-known for their ability to reverse gray hair. There is no suggested amount, but it should be incorporated into the daily diet, in soups, salads and breads. Black sesame seeds are commonly found at Asian markets.

Bhringaraja (bringaraj or eclipta alba) is often translated to mean "Hair King," It is a traditional

Ayurvedic herb native to the Himalayas, which is regarded as a rejuvenator and a liver and kidney tonic. It is a boon to the digestive system and strengthens the nervous system. In the East, it is widely credited with promoting hair health and reversing baldness and gray hair.

There are no established amounts to be taken for gray hair reversal, but 250 mg tablets are suggested twice per day (first thing upon awakening and at night before retiring to bed) as a liver tonic. It is available as a juice, oil, in tablets, powdered and as dried leaves, which may be made into a tea or tincture.

Fo-ti (he-shou-wu or polygonum multiflorum) is a Chinese herb whose name is translated to mean "black-haired Mr. He." It is widely credited with rejuvenating and anti-aging properties, including the restoration of natural hair color.

It is a tonic for the kidneys, the cardiovascular system, blood and liver. It promotes enhanced immune function, healthy tissues and glandular support. A commonly suggested amount is 3,000 to 6,000 mg in two to three divided doses, daily in capsules. It may, also, be taken as a tincture.

Caution: Mild gastrointestinal disturbances have been reported along with a rare potential liver reaction when using Fo-ti.

Ginger improves circulation, reduces anxiety and promotes relaxation. It is an an ingredient in many gray hair reversing remedies. It may be taken in capsules or in powdered form. The fresh root can, also, be juiced, made into tea or used in soups and a variety of other recipes.

For gray hair reversal, combine equal parts of fresh, grated ginger and raw honey. Consume 1 to 2 tsp. daily.

Moringa (moringa oleifera) is a flowering tree native to India and Africa. Its leaves are a powerful, rejuvenating superfood packed with the vitamins, minerals and enzymes commonly necessary to facilitate gray hair reversal. It is gaining popularity in the West where it is typically found in dried or capsule form. There is no recommended amount. It is not known to have any negative side effects.

Neem (margosa) leaves are commonly taken as a tea for a variety of conditions. It is regarded as a panacea and many studies on the powers of neem in its various forms have been conducted in India. It is beneficial to the skin and hair and is believed to reverse gray hair when it used consistently.

Red pine needle (pinus densiflora) is native to Japan. It is not an inexpensive remedy, but it has long been regarded as an anti-aging, rejuvenating remedy in Japan and Korea and is credited with returning gray hair to its natural color. It purifies the blood, stimulates the function of the thyroid gland, balances pH, protects from environmental pollutants including radiation, strengthen cells, increases oxygenation and improves overall health and energy levels. It can be found in oil and capsule form. Follow the directions on the bottle and heed all warnings. This remedy is not good for pregnant women.

Turmeric is a plant native to tropical South Asia, which contains the important constituent curcumin. It is a skin rejuvenator that been known to turn gray hair back to its natural color. It is, also, used as a natural dye to gradually turn gray hair blond. If you purchase supplements, follow the dosage recommendations on the bottle. Otherwise, try 1/4 to 1/2 tsp. twice per day in warm water.

A combination remedy is as follows: Combine equal parts of powdered amla, powdered neem leaves and turmeric. Take 1 tsp. daily with distilled water.

Thomas W. Xander

11 TOPICAL TREATMENTS FOR GRAY HAIR REVERSAL

Topical gray hair reversal treatments are another way for the body to absorb nutrients from oils, herbs and foods. They can be used in conjunction with oral remedies or alone.

A gentle, thorough massage of the hair and scalp with natural oils is a way to increase circulation and oxygenation while delivering nutrients to the place where they can be directly absorbed the hair and scalp.

For this purpose, different oils can be used either alone or in combination with others. The most popular is coconut oil, however, others include:

Almond oil
Black seed oil
Castor oil
Jojoba oil
Mustard seed oil
Milk thistle oil
Olive oil

Safflower oil

To one or two ounces of the above oils, add a few drops of any of the following essential oils (not fragrance oils) for more anti-graying power: Benzoin, cedarwood, ginger, lavender, lemon, neem, rosemary, sage, sandalwood, thyme and ylang-ylang. Store your custom oil concoction in a dark bottle, away from light and heat.

Use the above topical treatments nightly, applying them to the hair before retiring and rinsing them out upon awakening. If you are blessed, with a thick head of hair that, also, has a little coarser texture, you may be able to use an oil treatment as a hair dressing. Style your hair and leave the oils on your scalp until the next time you shampoo.

A special topical oil treatment for vitiligo is as follows: Coconut oil, psoralea seed (psoralea crolyforlia) oil, black cumin oil and barberry root extract. In China, psoralea is credited with reversing baldness and hair loss. These ingredients are available from online herb stores.

Mustard oil is a powerful treatment for gray hair that works very quickly for some people. Massage mustard oil on your hair nightly before going to bed and rinse it out in the morning. You may see results in as little as two weeks.

Amla (Indian gooseberry) crushed and mixed into coconut oil may help hair regain its natural color when it is applied to the scalp regularly. This is a well-known Indian remedy.

Crush amla seeds and add a little water to make a paste. Apply this to the hair overnight. Add power to this preparation with an equal part of crushed mango seeds.

Alternatively, combine equal parts of amla oil, coconut oil and lemon juice and apply this remedy to your scalp.

More Topical Remedies

Combine a tablespoon of black seed oil or coconut oil with a few drops of lemon juice and apply it to your scalp.

Rinse your hair daily with sage tea.

Boil some curry leaves in coconut oil. Cool, strain and apply the liquid to your scalp.

Apply amaranth leaf extract to the hair and scalp nightly. It is available from health food stores, some large grocery stores and online.

Argan oil is extracted from the seeds of an ancient Moroccan tree. It is a beauty oil of ancient fame, which is highly beneficial to the skin and hair. It is a natural anti-friz agent and a heat protectant. It, also, has a reputation for restoring hair color. It is not an inexpensive product, but a little goes a long way. A few drops may be rubbed into the hair, after washing and drying, as a conditioner and to guard against breakage.

Apply fresh onion juice to the scalp nightly.

Onion Juice Topical Remedy

Ramp up the power of your onion juice application as follows:

1 tsp. onion juice
1 tsp. lemon juice
1 tsp. almond oil
1/4 tsp. freshly ground black pepper

A few times per week, apply this mixture to your scalp and leave it for, at least, half an hour.

Black Pepper and Lemon Topical Remedy

1/8 tsp. freshly ground black pepper
1/2 cup yogurt
1/2 tsp. lemon juice
1/2 tsp. almond oil

Blend these ingredients thoroughly and apply this mixture to your hair and scalp. Leave it for half an hour before washing it out. Repeat this procedure twice per week to help restore natural hair color and prevent any further graying of hair.

12 NATURAL HAIR COLOR ENHANCERS (DYES)

If you still want to cover up a few gray hairs or enhance your natural hair color without the use of harsh chemicals, you may want to try one of the following natural colorants. While they are primarily dyes, some of them are very mild and they actually have health benefits for you hair and scalp. Although, most of these natural methods will not work well for people who have a lot of gray hair.

Henna is a common natural dye for all shades of red, brown and darker hair. Black henna or indigo is used for black or very dark hair. It is available at beauty supply stores, herb stores and Indian stores. Carefully follow any instructions that accompany your purchase. These are permanent dyes and their effects last about three months, so test a small, inconspicuous area, first. You should choose a shade of henna that closely matches your natural color. Henna will not lighten your hair.

Caution: Some people are sensitive to henna. Authentic, natural henna dyes should not contain chemical developers.

Non-henna treatments must be performed consistently for a while to see results. Teas may be placed into a spray bottle for easier application. During the application, you may apply a plastic cap or a piece of kitchen plastic wrap to your hair to keep warmth in and keep the application from drying out prematurely. Alternatively, wrap your hair in a warm towel to prolong the action for, at least, an hour or as long as possible unless the instructions state otherwise.

When using these substances, take the same precautions you would with any dyes where your clothes, carpeting, linoleum and towels are concerned to prevent stains. When working with henna, use plastic gloves. Henna will stain skin and anything else it comes in contact with.

Black Henna (Indigo) for Black Hair

Obtain organic, black henna, which is often ordinary henna combined with indigo or just indigo.

Combine black henna with water to create a paste of about the same consistency as yogurt. Apply it to your hair, covering it thoroughly from the roots to the end. Wrap your head in a towel and leave it for about half an hour. If you have any drips, wipe them away immediately, otherwise it will leave a stain on your skin.

Rinse it out of your hair. After a day or so, the hair will be very black.

Generally, short hair requires 2-3 oz. of henna; medium-length hair requires 3-5 oz.; and long hair requires 5-8 oz.

A Mild Dye for Black or Brown Hair

Make a tea of 1/2 tsp. dried stinging nettles, 1/2 tsp.

sage and 1/4 tsp. rosemary. Allow it to cool and use it as a rinse for your hair. Apply it after shampooing. Do not rinse it out.

Optionally, add Fo-ti to the above tea by emptying one or two capsules and adding it to the tea mixture.

Henna for Auburn and Red Hair

Red henna is the most popular natural dye for red hair. Follow the same instructions for black henna above.

A Mild Tea Dye for Reddish Shades

Make a strong tea or decoction with red hibiscus petals. Allow it to cool, strain it and apply it to your hair. Do not rinse it out.

For Blond Hair

Make a strong tea or decoction of turmeric and allow it to cool. Add a little bit of lemon juice and apply it to your hair. Do not rinse it out.

Other herbs used in teas for blond hair include: Chamomile, calendula, purple loose strife and fenugreek seeds.

Add a small amount of peroxide to your shampoo to keep lighter shades bright and discourage graying. This remedy can, also, be used on darker shades of hair, but it may cause unwanted lightening.

Thomas W. Xander

13 HOW TO USE RADIESTHESIA TO DETERMINE THE RIGHT REMEDY FOR YOU

If you've just finished reading about all of these remedies for reversing gray hair, you might be feeling a little overwhelmed. But, chances are you, also, felt some resonance with, at least, one or two of them.

If you've been jotting down notes as something you read struck you as particularly useful in your case, you may already know what kind of gray hair reversal regimen you would like to experiment with.

Your choices about remedies may involve accessibility to the ingredients. For example, if you don't live in a place where you have easy access to exotic grocery stores, you can experiment using more common foods and herbs. If you have allergies or other health conditions that preclude you from eating certain foods, of course, you will want to take that into consideration.

But, if you have any doubts about where to begin, you can resolve them through the use of medical radiesthesia. Despite its scientific-sounding name, using medical radiesthesia is a simple and fun exercise in self-exploration.

The following description and exercise for the employment of medical radiesthesia using a pendulum given below is extracted from the book, *Magical Healing: How to Use Your Mind to Heal Yourself and Others*, by Angela Kaelin.[8]

The term radiesthesia means "to perceive radiation" and it pertains to other forms of dowsing, however, in this exercise we will be using a simple pendulum. The term is often used in reference to medical dowsing, but it is sometimes used to refer to dowsing, in general.

The hypothesis of medical radiesthesia is that all things emit radiation; a current of energy flows through human hands; and objects can become tools by which to obtain information about a subject.

Basics of Using a Pendulum for Radiesthesia

It is best to acquire a pendulum that is properly weighted and balanced, but almost anything can be used as a pendulum. It is simply a weight suspended from a length of string or chain. You "tune" the pendulum by adjusting its length. A shorter length swings faster than a longer one. This is a matter of personal preference.

The pendulum appears to work on the basis of energy and impulses sent through the body as a result of directed thought.

Whenever you use a pendulum, you must formulate a question and then wait, with the attitude of an observer for the response.

A pendulum does not work exactly the same way for every person. There are two ways to determine pendulum indications for you:

The first is to simply ask the pendulum. Hold the

pendulum suspended in front of you and command it. Say, "Show me what 'yes' is for me." Then, wait and watch what the pendulum does. It may go in a clockwise or counter-clockwise circle, it may swing back and forth or it may remain still. This is your "Yes" indication.

Then command it to show you your "No" response. Say, "Show me what 'No' is for me." Then, wait and watch what the pendulum does. Again, it may go in a clockwise or counter-clockwise circle, it may swing back and forth or it may remain still. This is your "No" indication.

The second method is to program the pendulum to move as you want it to for certain indications. Commonly used indications are to have the pendulum swing back and forth for "Yes," from side to side for "No" and around in a circle when the question cannot be answered.

In medical radiesthesia, it is common to have the pendulum swing back and forth when it is "neutral," in a clockwise direction for "Yes" and in a counter-clockwise direction for "No."

Make these pendulum motions intentionally, at first. Practice like this for a few minutes.

Then, pause and with a serious mind test your pendulum by asking it a question you already know the answer to. For example, "Is my name _____?" Then, wait for the answer.

Hold the pendulum over a common object like a book and ask, "Is this a book?" Wait for the answer. Then, hold the pendulum over the same object and as, "Is this a rock?"

After you do this several times and receive consistently correct responses from the pendulum, it is programmed.

Determining the Right Remedy

Use the following list of remedies in this book to formulate your own dowsing charts. These can be pie-style charts or a simple list. To use a list, put your finger on the item or hold your pendulum over it and ask, "Is this the right remedy for me?"

For your radiesthesia to be effective, you must make a mental connection between yourself and the substance you are testing. You may write your name on the paper to help you remember that you are testing these remedies for yourself. Professionals use a "witness," which is a substance like a hair sample, recent photograph, saliva or blood droplet that represents the person.

Choose a quiet place to work where you can remain undisturbed for, at least, 15 or 20 minutes.

You may find it helpful to begin with the list of Possible Causes of Gray Hair.

Write all of the remedies relevant to you on a list. Place your finger on the remedy and ask the pendulum to answer the question: "Is this the right remedy to reverse my gray hair?"

Summary of Basic Gray Hair Remedies

Possible Causes of Gray Hair

Adrenal fatigue
Thyroid imbalance
Toxic burden
Poor circulation
Vitiligo
Nutritional deficiencies

Detoxification

Oil pulling

Vitamins

Vitamin A
B-complex
Vitamin B1
Vitamin B2
Vitamin B3
Vitamin B5
Vitamin B6
Vitamin B7
Vitamin B9
Vitamin B12
Inositol
Choline
PABA
Vitamin C
Vitamin E

Minerals

Copper
Zinc
Manganese
Magnesium
Iodine (Note: Use radiesthesia to see if your thyroid is over-functioning, under-functioning or balanced. Afterward, if necessary, test for the right remedies.)

Blackstrap Molasses

Unsulphured blackstrap molasses
Regimen #1 Blackstrap Molasses Anti-gray Hair Drink

Regimen #2 Blackstrap Molasses Anti-gray Hair Drink
Regimen #3 Blackstrap Molasses Anti-gray Hair Drink
Regimen #4 Blackstrap Molasses, Vitamin and Mineral
Combination
Regimen #5 Blackstrap Molasses pH Balancing

Enzymes from Raw and Fermented Foods

Cabbage
Carrots
Beets
Celery
Daikon radishes
Dark leafy green vegetables
Fenugreek seed sprouts (are a stand-alone remedy for
some cases of gray hair)
White (Irish) potatoes (provide the enzyme catalase, a
deficiency of which is implicated in gray hair)
Sour apples including the peeling (also, provide catalase)
Wheatgrass (high in chlorophyll, contains many anti-
gray hair vitamins and minerals)
Mulberries (a kidney tonic)
All fruits and dark berries
Raw honey
Raw dairy products
Apple cider vinegar
Kombucha tea
Miso (soybean curd)
Yogurt
Kefir
Sourdough breads which are homemade, preferably with
whole grains.

Essential Fatty Acids

Black seed oil (black cumin or nigella sativa) is a

legendary Indian anti-gray hair remedy.
Chia seeds are a superfood credited with anti-aging and overall all health benefits.
Flax seed (crushed or oil) Flax seed oil must be refrigerated and should not be heated in cooking.
Fish oil.
Sesame seeds
Seaweed
Wheat germ oil
DHA

Blood and Kidney Tonics

Asparagus
Beets
Carrots
Blackstrap molasses
Black sesame seeds
Chlorophyll
Cranberries
Cucumbers
Dandelion roots
Hyssop
Nettles
Parsley
Seaweed
Strawberry leaves
Watermelon seeds as a tea
Wheatgrass

Common Remedies

Chlorophyll
Irish (White) Potato
Citrus peeling (Vitamin C)
Resveratol

Lemons
Onions
Chia seeds

Asian Remedies

Amla (Indian gooseberry)
Black seed (nigella or black cumin)
Black sesame seeds
Bhringaraja
Fo-ti (He-Shou-Wu)
Ginger
Moringa
Neem (Margosa)
Red pine needle
Turmeric

Topical Treatments for Gray Hair Reversal

Almond oil
Black seed oil
Castor oil
Jojoba oil
Mustard seed oil
Milk thistle oil
Olive oil
Benzoin
Cedarwood
Ginger
Lavender
Lemon
Neem
Psoralea seed (psoralea crolyforlia) oil
Rosemary
Safflower oil
Sage

Sandalwood
Thyme
Ylang-ylang

Vitiligo Topical Remedy: Coconut, psoralea seed, black cumin and barberry root
Argan oil

Once you have determined the right remedies, use the pendulum to determine the proper daily dosage for you. Where recommendations have been given in the book, begin with that amount and ask if it is right for you. If the answer given is, "No," then ask if you need more or less. Then, in increments ask, "Is this the right amount?" until you get a "Yes" answer.

Caution: Use common sense and reason when finding amounts, especially with regard to vitamin supplements. Taking too much of some vitamin supplements for long periods of time may lead to liver damage.

You may, also, use radiesthesia to determine how long a particular remedy will take to show results for you. Begin by asking the pendulum, "Will I see positive results from this remedy in two weeks?" If the answer is "No," then incrementally increase the amount of time and formulate the question again. "Will I see positive results from this remedy in three weeks?" If the answer is "No," then continue on in this fashion until you reach a "Yes" response.

Radiesthesia, more commonly called "dowsing," with pendulums, rods, twigs and bobbers has long been used to find water, minerals, hidden treasure, lost objects and missing people. It is a very natural thing to do, but the ability has been lost or blocked by many people because of the prevalence of superstitious religious beliefs.

You should be able to pick this ability up in a matter of minutes, but if you would like to learn more about dowsing, contact the American Society of Dowsers, which is a nationwide organization that teaches people how to dowse. (www.dowsers.org) A similar organization exists in the U.K. (www.britishdowsers.org)

REFERENCES

1. Trinidad, P. Trinidad, Ph. D., Aida C. Mallillin, Rosario S. Sagum, PhD., Rosario R. Encabo. Zolio B. Villanueva, "Glycemic Index of Coco Sugar," Republic of the Philippines, Department of Science and Technology, Food and Nutrition Research Institute. http://www.pca.da.gov.ph/pdf/glycemic.pdf

2. Blaylock, Russell L. "Excitotoxins: The Taste that Kills," Health Press, December 1, 1996.

3. Montes LF, Diaz ML, Lajous J, Garcia NJ., "Folic acid and vitamin B12 in vitiligo: a nutritional approach," Department of Dermatology, University of Alabama, Birmingham Medical Center. Cutis. 1992 Jul;50(1):39-42.

4. Juhlin, L and MJ Olson. "Improvement of vitiligo after oral treatment with vitamin B12 and folic acid and the importance of sun exposure," Department of Dermatology, University Hospital, Uppsala, Sweden.

Acta Derm Venereol. 2002;82(5):369-72.

5. Edgar Cayce's Association for Research and Enlightenment.
www.edgarcayce.org/IntSearchHealthDatabase/data/thca lcio.html?terms=gray%20hair

6. Wood, JM, Decker H, Hartmann H, Chavan B, Rokos H, Spencer JD, Hasse S, Thornton MJ, Shalbaf M, Paus R, Schallreuter KU. "Senile hair graying: H2O2-mediated oxidative stress affects human hair color by blunting methionine sulfoxide repair," Clinical and Experimental Dermatology/Department of Biomedical Sciences, University of Bradford, Bradford, BD7 1DP, West Yorkshire, UK. FASEB J. 2009 Jul;23(7):2065-75. Epub 2009 Feb 23. Retrieved on January 20, 2012. http://www.ncbi.nlm.nih.gov/pubmed?term=catalayse %20peroxide%20gray%20hair

7. Floreani, Maura, Eleonora Napoli, Luigi Quintieri, Pietro Palatini,."Oral administration of trans-resveratrol to guinea pigs increases cardiac DT-diaphorase and catalase activities, and protects isolated atria from menadione toxicity," Department of Pharmacology and Anesthesiology, University of Padova, Largo Meneghetti 2, 35131 Padova, Italy, Life Sciences, Volume 72, Issue 24, 2 May 2003, Pages 2741-2750 Retrieved 1/21/2012. http://dx.doi.org/10.1016/S0024-3205(03)00179-6

8. Kaelin, Angela. "Magical Healing: How to Use Your Mind to Heal Yourself and Others," Winter Tempest Books, 2011.

OTHER WINTER TEMPEST BOOKS

If you enjoyed this book, you might enjoy other Winter Tempest Books:

Magical Healing: How to Use Your Mind to Heal Yourself and Others by Angela Kaelin

All Natural Dental Remedies: Herbs and Home Remedies to Heal Your Teeth and Naturally Restore Tooth Enamel by Angela Kaelin

Traditional Witches' Formulary and Potion-making Guide: Recipes for Magical Oils, Powders and Other Potions by Sophia diGregorio

Legal Disclaimer: The author and publisher of this guide has used his or her best efforts in preparing this document. The author makes no representation or warranties with respect to the accuracy, applicability, fitness or completeness of the contents of this document. The author disclaims any warranties expressed or implied. Nothing in this document should be construed as medical advice. The author shall in no event be held liable for any loss or damages, including but not limited to special, incidental, consequential or other damages incurred by the use of this information. The statements in this book have not been evaluated by the F.D.A., the A.M.A., the A.D.A. or any other government organization. The statements contained herein represent the legally protected opinions of the author and are presented for informational purposes only. If anyone uses any of this information in the book, they do so at their own risk. This document contains material protected under copyright laws. Any unauthorized reprint, transmission or resale of this material without the express permission of the author is strictly prohibited.

FTC Disclaimer: The author has no connection to nor was paid by any brand or product described in this document except for Winter Tempest Books.

FDA Disclaimer: The statements in this book are the opinion of the author and have not been evaluated by the Food and Drug Administration. Products and information provided on this site are not intended to diagnose, treat, cure or prevent any disease. If you have a medical condition, consult your physician. All information is provided for educational purposes only. Please consult your doctor if your pregnant. Keep these and all supplements out of the reach of children.